Ripples f

CU00822422

Althea Hayton

Wren Publications

First published in 2014 by
Wren Publications
PO Box 396
St Albans
Herts
AL3 6NE
England

Copyright ©Althea Hayton 2014

"Ripples" cover image by Monica Hudson

ISBN 978-0-9557808-8-2

Printed and bound in UK and USA by Lightning Source:
Lightning Source UK
Chapter House, Pitfield, Kiln Farm Milton Keynes
Bucks, MK11 3LW, UK

Lightning Source Inc (US)
1246 Heil Quaker Blvd.
La Verne, TN, USA, 37086

CONTENTS

ACKNOWLEDGEMENTS

This little book has taken many years to develop and would not have been possible to create without the help of many hundreds of people across the world - and five people in particular.

First of all, my thanks to the many hundreds of womb twin survivors who over the last decade have responded to the various questionnaires and sent me their stories. Their patience and willingness to take part in the research has enabled us to produce some good and reliable data.

Thanks to the hundreds of womb twin survivors who have trusted me enough to enter into a deeper exploration of their feelings, mainly by email. It has been a great privilege to be part of their journey.

Special thanks to the five therapists who came together with me earlier this year to create this manual. Thank you to Monica Hudson, Pamela and Tyrone Lester, Alfred Ramoda Austermann and Andrew Griffin.

Finally, a big Thank You to Celeste Hardingham, who helped with the proof reading but especially because, as Chairman of Womb Twin, she will take this work into the future.

Althea Hayton June 2014

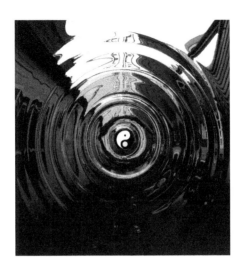

Introduction

This manual is a beginner's guide to the womb twin work, which is a specific set of therapeutic interventions which are known to be helpful for womb twin survivors. The ideas, advice and explanations provided here will help you to notice any womb twin survivors among your clients and provide them with appropriate help and guidance as they follow their healing path.

A womb twin survivor is an individual who started life in the womb as a twin, but their twin died before or around birth. The term is also used to describe the sole survivor of a multiple pregnancy (i.e. triplets or more.) Since the launch of the womb twin survivors research project in 2003, various resources for womb twin survivors of all ages, and their parents, have been created.

It has taken many years to gain sufficient perspective on the psychological effects experienced by womb twin survivors to be able to create this simple manual for therapists of all disciplines.

[Please note that this manual does not cover the background biology, details of the healing path or full references. If you wish to benefit fully from this manual in order to learn how to identify womb twin survivors among your present and future clients and offer them appropriate help, you will need to do some background reading.]

We begin with the biggest problem: recognising the possibility that a particular client may be a womb twin survivor. Womb twin survivors do not always know that they once had a twin. Alternatively, they may know but not realise that there can be any consequent psychological effects. It may fall to the therapist to make that clear.

To explain the reality of the pre-natal loss of a twin to a client requires a good understanding of the physical and psychological characteristics of womb twin survivors. This manual provides some basic details. Once the twin is accepted as a reality, then the way in which the client lives out the deep imprint of the loss of their twin - which is not the same as a definite memory but has a dream-like quality - can be explored in depth. This is known to be highly therapeutic for womb twin survivors.

The individual response to the loss of a twin or more can badly affect the life of the womb twin survivor. There is a tendency towards self-defeating behaviour, which makes the therapy very difficult, or even impossible, to continue.

The relationship with the twin that is made in the womb is the first-ever relationship in the life of the womb twin survivor. It becomes the template for all other relationships in born life. The nature of that relationship template can be discovered and explored in the therapeutic encounter. The therapist can become a surrogate twin. Despite the comfort and satisfaction this brings, it can stall any therapeutic progress, as we will see.

Regardless of the style of therapy being used, the womb twin work can usefully include rituals of various kinds, related to a pre-natal experience of loss. Rituals may be beyond the usual methods of working for some therapists, so some examples of rituals that are known to be helpful are described.

The womb twin work can be excessively prolonged by a high level of resistance in the client. This becomes apparent after a while, when no appreciable improvement is seen, despite a huge effort being made by the therapist. Healing is a choice, and some womb twin survivors, owing to a high level of survivor guilt, cannot allow themselves to heal.

The healing begins only when the client makes a resolution to choose life and live life to the full. Existential issues - life, death, choice, responsibility - are an important feature of this stage. Despite the fact that the client has been willingly showing up to do the work, they still need to make this choice if the next healing stage is to be achieved.

The womb twin work is done when the client experiences revival and becomes more alive, more effective and more positive. The process of the womb twin work having been completed, the original presenting problem, if not already solved by the womb twin work, can be worked on more effectively. (Eg. addictions, compulsions, marital difficulties, prolonged grief etc.) Thus, the womb twin work is not a replacement for therapy, but a useful starting point if your client is a womb twin survivor. It can be a way to get to the root source of your client's pain.

At the time of writing, there are only a few systems of therapy that routinely include the concept of the pre-natal loss of a twin. As awareness of the special psychology of womb twin survivors spreads across the profession, therapists and healers across a wide spectrum of modalities will begin to adapt the womb twin work to fit comfortably with their usual way of working.

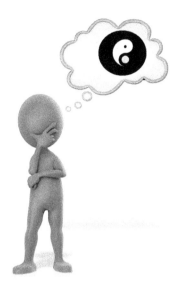

Recognition

Womb twin survivors are different from other clients, but the differences are subtle and hard to identify. Thanks to the womb twin survivors research project, we now have a reliable psychological profile for womb twin survivors.[1,2] We also now know much more about the physical signs and indications of a twin or multiple pregnancy that resulted in only one live birth.

You can begin the process of finding out whether or not a client is a womb twin survivor in three simple ways:

Checklists
The client can complete a checklist as part of the initial assessment. There are two checklists that can be used: (*see appendix.*)

- A list of the physical signs and indications that there had been twins or more at some stage in the mother's pregnancy.

- A list of the twenty most common psychological traits found among womb twin survivors.

  One client said to me one day, "I wish you were my twin." I thought at the time that it was a little odd, but I didn't know then about womb twin survivors.

Key words

Certain words with a deeper meaning may be repeated often and emphasised, particularly in the very first session:

- Related to death, grief or bereavement
- Related to being alone, rejected or aban-doned
- Related to being different, odd or weird

Ways of relating

For womb twin survivors, the way they formed a bond with their twin can become the template for their intimate relationships.

For example:

- Trying to merge with the other person
- Not allowing a relationship to develop
- Treating everyone like a sibling, regardless of social rank

  In Susan's family constellation, her two representatives, one for her and one for a missing person, were entwined in an endless embrace, both smiling dreamily. I said "It is like you have found your twin," Susan burst into tears, but she was smiling broadly.

Knowing and not knowing

Some people are womb twin survivors but have no idea that this could be the case. Others have been told, but do not realise that the pre-natal loss of a twin can have a psychological effect. Still others may have been told of their twin and are in full awareness of the effects of the loss, but they hesitate to mention it, lest the idea be dismissed as unimportant.

Reassessment of previous clients

When you have had some experience of discovering womb twin survivors among your new clients, it may be possible to review your work with previous clients, to see whether or not they are womb twin survivors.

They may have been unconsciously trying to tell you about their twin for a long time, but you did not realise the significance. They may even describe their sense of the dynamics of different personalities in their inner world, but a connection to the womb experience may not have been made.

They may have spoken openly about the fact they they were once a twin, but you overlooked it, not understanding what it meant.

During the previous work with a client, a pattern may be detected that suggests prenatal twinning. One example could be a pattern of too-close relationships that are deliberately cut short before they can fully develop.

As your suspicions begin to mount that a particular client is a womb twin survivor, you could consider bringing this possibility into the therapy. There are many ways to do this.

On the whole, it seems to be good practice not to simply say, "I think you are a womb twin survivor." Rather, it is probably better to hint at it in various ways and let the client find the idea in his or her own way.

Broaching the subject to a client

Broaching the subject to a client at any stage in their therapy is best done with great sensitivity. The loss of a twin before birth is experienced in many different ways by the sole survivors. Research has shown that this aspect of the subject makes it very hard to pin down, or explain to clients who have never come across it before.

One person may be elated and relieved to find the final piece of the puzzle, whereas another may be plunged almost immediately into a "Black hole" of depression and loss. It is not possible to know in advance how the news of this possibility will be received.

Some clients, even if they know they are womb twin survivors, may simply not be ready to talk about it. Others may be completely unmoved by the idea. If the whole idea is beyond your normal scope of practice, this may be enough to keep you silent on the subject.

Halfway through the session he asked, 'So what do you think is the root cause of all your pain?' I thought about this and said, 'Probably the fact that I was adopted, that I was actually abandoned at birth.' His reply was, 'That's not it; it is earlier than that.' I thought some more and tentatively said, 'It must have been due to the horrible feelings and emotions I felt living in the womb of my birth mother.' His reply again was, 'No, that is not it.' That surprised me and my next thought was, 'Bloody hell, please don't tell me this is due to some past life stuff.' Having worked on plenty of past life stuff before, I saw no solution in that. He asked me, 'Are you ready to hear this? Do you want to know the real cause?' I looked at him and firmly said, 'Yes'.

He said, 'You are a womb twin survivor. You had a twin in the womb who died.' This shocked me. I had never heard of this before. At the same time what I was hearing actually felt familiar. Of course I had no proof but as we talked about it and he brought me through a questionnaire, based on the symptoms and characteristics of womb twin survivors, I appeared to be a textbook example.

Apparently the loss of my twin in the womb had a severe energetic and psychological impact on me and since then I was living life in a post-traumatic stress state. This seemed bizarre but I was relieved that I had possibly reached the beginning of the end of my pain.

However, the deep wisdom that is in every client will dictate how fast or slow the therapy moves forward. It can be very frustrating if you as the therapist realise that a certain client is a womb twin survivor, which fully explains their deep distress and unhappiness, only to find that the client doesn't want to know. For many womb twin survivors, resistance to healing is very strong, as we shall see.

Seeing the first therapist was really good. He allowed me to talk freely about things, asking if my twin was a boy or girl. He was just matter of fact, and allowed me to accept being a twin as the truth. I couldn't afford further sessions so I switched to another therapist. I didn't find him as easy as the first. He suggested I need to accept that it's likely I'll never know the truth.

Bearing in mind these difficulties, there are three ways to broach the subject.

1. Gently suggest it in general terms: "It looks like some of these problems began before you were born."

2. Use the assessment checklists: "I have some new assessment materials that you may like to see."

3. Seize the opportunity to gently mention the possibility, if the client seems to be very close to the idea. In family constellation groups, the lost twin sometimes emerges as a missing family member, who can then be gently identified.

4. The checklist of psychological effects can be used in various ways, particularly if a client knows about their twin but has not yet made the connection between that loss and their psychological make-up.

Therapists speak from experience

• *Some womb twin survivors pick up feelings from someone else, due to having poor boundaries. It may feel as if unresolved spirits latch onto/infect them. They may continue to believe this for a lifetime, until the truth is uncovered.*

- *Hold your intention to explore, stay open, look for subtler layers that may be something else.*

- *Some people are blind to being a womb twin survivor and wish to remain so, but the therapist can gradually work on the associated issues until they are ready to explore the idea.*

- *If a client is suicidal and they show enough signs and indications to convince you that they may be a womb twin survivor, it may be worth speaking out at an earlier stage, for it could save their life.*

- *Knowledge of pre-birth effects on relationships alters one's perspective on the role of parents in developing a child's personality. The pre-natal loss of a twin can lead to self isolation, making it very hard for parents to establish a good relationship with their child.*

- *In family constellations, twinning doesn't always appear immediately. In the more classic style of constellations, how quickly the twin is "found" depends very much on the objectives of the person and the ability of the constellator to relate symptoms to it. It is crucial for the therapist to evaluate if the person is a womb twin survivor or not. If that is not correctly considered, working on other systemic areas of the patient could lead to more frustration, because no final answers are found.*

References

1. www.wombtwinsurvivors.com
2. Hayton, A. *A healing path for womb twin survivors,* Wren Publications 2012

Twin pregnancy at 8 weeks

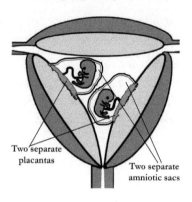

Two separate placantas

Two separate amniotic sacs

Reality

Womb twin survivors seem to spend their lives re-enacting the life and death of their womb twin. Nothing appears to be more important than that, even life itself. But once the real pre-birth scene, which is being constantly re-enacted, is made clear, the re-enactment tends to diminish or cease altogether, greatly to the benefit of the individual.

The process of therapy, therefore, necessarily includes an attempt to unravel the vague impression of life in the womb. This has been called the "Dream of the Womb" because it is not a memory like other memories, but has a dream-like quality, which makes it very hard to attribute to anything real. Even for womb twin survivors themselves, the idea of some kind of pre-birth memory/ imprint can seem impossible, despite that fact that they often have a strong intuitive sense of their twin.

As the therapist listens to the story, the constant re-enactment of the pre-birth scene, (i.e. the presence of another or others, the death and absence of the twin) appears in every aspect of the therapy:

- The story of the twin as eventually worked out by the womb twin survivor.
- Echoes of the twin story in whatever is spoken about with the therapist or in the group.
- The relationship to the therapist and/or group members.
- The client's other close relationships as discussed in the sessions.
- The attitude the womb twin survivor has to being alive.
- The meta-narrative: the effect on the therapist; what is not told - the shame, the success, the contradictions.

What actually happened?

How much does the client know about the reality of their womb twin?

An important precursor to the womb twin work is to recognise the reality of the pre-natal imprint/memory. This lies deep down in the unconscious. If there is no factual knowledge of the twin anywhere in the family, then both client and therapist must rely on intuition, backed up by a conviction that the intuitive sense, although never perfect, is an excellent indicator of what lies in the unconscious.

For people who may be womb twin survivors, it is right to remain sceptical about what appears to be the truth. However, as the exploration continues, more and more clues may be revealed, in which case it will become increasingly difficult to prove oneself wrong in believing that one is a womb twin survivor.

Questions to answer:
- Did the womb twin develop a body at all (dermoid cyst, chimera, extra fingers or toes)
- At what point did the womb twin stop developing?
- Why did the womb twin die?
- When did the womb twin die?
- Who knows about the womb twin?
- Is there any proof that a womb twin once existed?

I am new to the womb twin world but it feels like coming home and a place where I can finally emerge in my wholeness, but I don't feel like anything done before has been in vain. It is all a part of me.

Homework for both client and therapis
- Look at images of twin pregnancies.
- Explore the intuitive sense of the possible nature of the womb twin (male, female, normal, abnormal etc.)
- Examine images of foetuses at different stages to see if any particular stage resonates with the intuitive sense of the womb twin.
- Watch slide shows, presentations, videos.
- Read stories by womb twin survivors on the internet or in a book.

Affirming the client's prebirth story
In the absence of proof, where there is some physical indication or strong psychological characteristic that can be identified, the client may come back to this again and again. While this may not be absolute proof, it can give

the client something to hold onto, as they try and piece their pre-birth story together.

There is no risk in affirming a client's feeling that they once had a twin. Experience has shown that only rarely do individuals latch on to the idea as the source of all their pain and distress, when in fact it is not true for them. If a client begins to use this explanation spuriously, they remain stuck, negative and static. If they truly are womb twin survivors, they will inevitably start moving, albeit sometimes rather slowly, along the healing path to a better life.

It took about three years to get the whole story straight. It was revealed to me bit by bit. It was like putting a ten thousand piece jigsaw puzzle together. I probably only have a thousand pieces in place, but that is enough for me. I am a womb twin survivor and my life has been completely transformed by this understanding.

Therapists speak from experience

- *I do think womb twin survivors need specific treatment. I've spent years dealing with my issues, and nothing really cleared because my issues were just a pattern, not the core.*

- *I recently worked with a mother and daughter together - the daughter radiated the symptoms and was utterly shocked when her mother told her that there was a small dead twin in the afterbirth when she was born.*

- *Ordinary psychotherapy that does not include the possibility of a twin loss does not hit the mark, can sometimes even torture the clients with wrong concepts and even reinforce an inherent tendency towards failure.*

- *Therapists need more information about intrauterine twin/triplet loss symptoms. They need the understanding that rational/cognitive talks are not sufficient to touch and heal the deep existential traumas. They also need the knowledge about other topics from the family system that interfere with the intrauterine/after birth loss of a twin.*

- *A big problem is not knowing they are womb twin survivors or not knowing what that meant and how it affects clients. In the famous words of Dr. Phil, "You cannot change what you do not acknowledge". Knowing was the biggest relief for me. The major problem is the lack of information and support for clients, especially in other languages.*

- *I had a friend, who at the age of 65 had an imaging done and found out she had three ureters and an extra small kidney. I could see in her behaviour that she was a womb twin survivor, but it had little or no impact on her beyond it being an anomaly. It would be interesting to know how common reabsorption and duplication occurs in the loss process but many may never know whether they have more than the normal numbers of parts. Someone else had an extra rib and another had two tailbones. I believe these are all signs of twin reabsorption, rather than cell division problems as they are developing.*

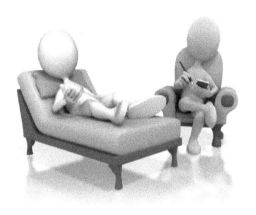

Relationship

In the kind of therapy where there are several sessions, a relationship begins to develop between therapist and client. There is much to be learned from how the relationship develops. It cannot be emphasised often enough that the bond that forms in the womb between twins - or more - becomes a template for all other close relationships in born life, as the re-enactment of the pre-natal story continues.

When working with womb twin survivors, it is vital to keep this in mind and to be aware of how the client is attempting to alter the professional relationship to fit with their Dream of the Womb. In short, the therapist in a sense "becomes" the missing twin in the mind of the client.

Children - and some adults - can make their own surrogate twin in the form of a soft toy or Teddy bear, but many of them will simply choose you, their therapist.

Alpha and Beta

In a twin pregnancy, even if the twins are identical, there is always one (the Alpha twin) who is better developed than the other (the Beta twin) even if it is by the tiniest margin. When both twins survive birth and grow to adulthood, that slight dominance of one over the other still remains. If the pregnancy is at all compromised and one twin dies, most of the time it is the Alpha twin who will survive.

Womb twin survivors are mostly - but not invariably - the Alpha twin of the pair. However, to keep their twin alive in their life they may unconsciously adopt some of the characteristics of their own Beta twin. (Eg. Being very strong and potentially healthy but refusing to practice self-care and thereby becoming weakened.) Now it is very important for therapists to be aware of this effect on the professional relationship. As the womb twin survivor attempts to keep their Dream of the Womb alive, they find ingenious ways to be both themselves and their twin in the same moment - Alpha and Beta.

Having two different sides to one's character is very common among womb twin survivors. In individual or group therapy the two sides may be represented in an exercise by two spaces, say either side of a line on the floor.

The movement from Alpha to Beta and back again can be very hard for some womb twin survivors. If they are stuck in their Beta space, they may turn you, their therapist, into their own Alpha twin. They will then allow you to lead and they will follow and obediently comply with your instructions – but not own decisions for themselves. This subtle and often overlooked effect can have a negative effect on the professional relationship.

It is important to leave the client on their own to take responsibility for their own healing – which for them may be the first glimmerings of what Alpha power is about. Your client will try every trick in the book to get you to tell them what to do next, but it is important to resist the impulse to lead and become the Alpha to their Beta. If it does happen that you end up encouraging and making suggestions, it is worth using the experience to discuss what is happening.

The client may realise that they can own their Alpha power for themselves if you wait - possibly for a very long time - while they turn up faithfully for every session or group meeting but do not let anything happen to further their own healing. This kind of passive, torpid client may already be familiar to you: if so, then it may help to discover if he or she is a womb twin survivor, and if so, explain about Alpha and Beta twins.

Maintaining separation

Your client may not be the only womb twin survivor in the room: With their finely-tuned empathy and intuition, many womb twin survivors become therapists. There is a possibility that you too may be a womb twin survivor. If so, it is important that you do your own womb twin work as soon as you can, or you risk becoming enmeshed in the issues of any womb twin survivor who may come to you for therapy. You are advised to find a therapist who can help you to discover the truth for yourself, join a process group or follow a published self-help plan, such as the Healing Path For Womb Twin Survivors.

If you have identified your own response to the loss of your womb twin, you will be able to remain separate from your client's process as the womb twin work continues.

Before I underwent my own healing process as a womb twin survivor, it was difficult to me to manage the bond with the womb twin survivors who were participants in the group.

Empathic failure

For some womb twin survivors and particularly, it seems, for the sole survivors of a one-egg twin pregnancy, a lack of empathy on the part of the therapist is experienced by the client as extremely painful, if not abusive, and certainly unprofessional.

One-egg twins do seem to have an extremely empathic relationship with each other that is unspoken, and can border on the telepathic. An identical twin would define empathetic failure as an extreme form of disappointment. This seems to be so with some clients, particularly those who are most resistant to change. In this case an extremely accurate kind of empathy is expected and anticipated, but of course cannot be provided, as the therapist is not clairvoyant.

Empathetic failure is described by some clients as the primary cause of their depression. In this case it is invariably an intimately related figure - parent, sibling or sexual partner - who has failed to display a sufficient level of empathy and this has caused great pain to the client. If the pain is related to the loss of a twin - the one person who could provide that level of empathy - then this response would make perfect sense.

In the absence of a highly empathetic, deeply-connected style of relationship, such as many therapists enjoy with their clients, then the client concerned reacts with pain, disappointment and resentment at the failure of the therapeutic relationship. After much struggle and a great deal of supervision for the therapist, the relationship ends - not without some tinge of relief for the therapist, who is left feeling exhausted and questioning their effectiveness.

Twin transference
In psychoanalysis, the desire by the client to make the analyst into a twin has been variously construed. (2) Because of the lack of knowledge of intrauterine events at the time when psychoanalytic theories were being formed, even until the 1980s and the advent of ultrasound scans, the possibility that this need may refer to a real missing twin was not considered.

Rescue
Womb twin survivors tend to have a strong rescue instinct, probably related to being the Alpha survivor. In close relationships the other person becomes the weaker, Beta twin, who must be saved.

Enmeshment
Womb twin survivors need you, their therapist, to merge with them - or at least, some of them do. This is potentially destructive of the professional relationship. If merging is allowed to happen, intentionally or not, then steps must be taken to back off without awakening abandonment /rejection trauma in the client.

If that also happens, then the trauma has to be worked through - all of which may prove overwhelming for the client.

Womb twin survivors are different

The discussion so far will have made it clear how different womb twin survivors are from other people. Furthermore, it has to be remembered that, in their constant search for the answer to why their client is so distressed, therapists who are not womb twin survivors themselves may categorise womb twin survivors as "disordered" or even "mentally ill."

Once a womb twin survivor has been labelled as having some kind of "personality disorder" then they have to go to great lengths to prove that after all, they are completely sane.

One famous case of misdiagnosis is that of Janet Frame, the famous New Zealand poet. Her identical twin died unnamed, two weeks after their birth, in 1924. Janet was labelled as schizophrenic as a teenager and spent eight years in mental hospital, narrowly missing being given a lobotomy. Many years later, having come across the world to London, she was reassessed at the Maudesly hospital and found to be completely sane.

The womb twin research project has revealed that many of the indications of "Borderline Personality Disorder" are also to be found among the most characteristic statements made by womb twin survivors who have physical evidence of their missing twin.

This strongly indicates that, if you have a client who shows all the signs of Borderline Personality Disorder, it may be worth using the checklists to establish whether or not they are womb twin survivors - if they are, they may have been misdiagnosed.

The womb twin work doesn't fit traditional paradigms, but womb twin survivors are normal. They are having a normal experience for a person with different sensitivities, and a pre-birth experience that only affects about 10% of the population. This means that 90% of the population, which would include medical professionals, do not understand this.

It is vitally important that therapists and other professionals learn how to identify womb twin survivors in any population so that appropriate treatment and support can be given.

They diagnosed me "schizophrenic" and "psychotic." Despite the fact that I was diagnosed as such, I had the feeling that something else was going on but I didn't know what that could be. I went back to school when I left the hospital. It was a very hard time. Every day I had to find a good reason to get out of bed and to go to school. For many years I felt very tired. I went for psychotherapy. Over the first years I saw many psychologists and psychiatrists. None of them could tell me what exactly was going on with me. I didn't get the answers I was so badly craving. I quit therapy several times over the years. I went back for therapy every time I started a new relationship, because then I was confronted again with something that was still wrong, but I couldn't put my finger on exactly what it was.. After four years of taking medication, I quit. I decided I could do it on my own. I didn't need it anymore. I haven't taken any medication since...........I recognised myself completely in the description of a womb twin survivor. I immediately started the 'womb twin work'. Only after two weeks of doing this work I started to feel much better and I was growing stronger day by day.

Therapists speak from experience

- *Womb twin survivors are often feeling guilty. They lack life power and energy. There is an immense longing for something. In their relationships they are either being very "melting" with partners, which can be too much for the other, or avoiding any kind of close contact at all. Often they lack money, for they feel they do not deserve the right to have a good job, house, relationship, to be happy in life.*

- *Vanishing twin diagnoses are rarely supported by factual evidence and vanishing twin symptoms are quite similar to siblings of an aborted foetus or miscarriages. We have worked with this issue for more than a hundred people, if entangled abortions are included - I'm often uncertain whether it's a vanished twin or an entangled abortion.*

- *The attraction between womb twin survivors (known or unknown) can be irresistible. A therapist who discovers they are a womb twin survivor and then meets a client who also is one, can be overwhelmed with feelings of connection and the need to merge. The recognition between them can be so exhilarating that it can easily overshadow the client- therapist relationship.*

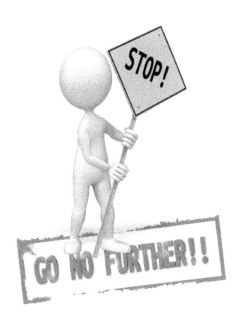

Resistance

The saddest and most frustrating aspect of therapy with womb twin survivors is the very high level of resistance to healing that can sometimes arise. Self-sabotage is very common among womb twin survivors, who willingly pursue a wide variety of healing therapies, one after the other, only to sabotage each of them in some way :

- Pretend to be healed and stop therapy
- Reject and decry the therapy style
- Complain about the therapist
- Manipulate the therapist into believing that healing is still possible, by allowing small, sporadic, short-lived improvements, soon reversed
- Remain silent about being a womb twin survivor

- Miss appointments and never explain why
- Just stop coming, with no reason given
- Try so hard to heal that healing is not allowed to occur

Healing is a choice

It is quite clear when we consider resistance that the progress of healing is firmly under the control of the client. The therapist can only guide those who have already chosen to take the healing path.

Healing cannot be hurried - or even encouraged - by the therapist. Even the most charismatic and inspiring healer will only bring about small, temporary changes, unless the client makes his or her own choice to begin the healing journey.

Existential issues

Death and non-life frequently appear as (possibly hidden) themes in therapy with womb twin survivors. Many clients have a problem with the fact their twin had no life, but they did. It seems unfair.

> *The one thing I have never been able to address in any therapeutical setting has been my deep longing to be removed from this earth. I'm not suicidal, however I long to be reunited (with my wt's?)... I have always been nostalgic of death and very connected to the energies of death/birth, even as a child.*

One way to even up the score, as it were, would be to choose not to have a life. This choice underpins resistance to healing. Womb twin survivors tend to sabotage their own therapy, despite paying a significant proportion of their income upon it.

There are many ways to be alive but not to have a life - e.g.. to live with diminished life force:

- Being unable to make choices
- Not taking responsibility
- Having no willpower
- Trying to live two lives at once
- Addiction
- Compulsive behaviour
- Feeling dead inside
- Disengaged - on the edge of life
- Dissociated - escape to an inner world
- Not realising true potential
- Lack of rest and self-care
- Lack of vitality due to unhealthy lifestyle
- Lack of assertiveness

I found out when I was twelve that my twin was stillborn. I felt guilty for a long time, then I felt I had to fill my life with as much experience as possible. This only served to ruin my life, looking for love and acceptance and making more than double my share of mistakes.

Why refuse life?

It is impossible to persuade someone who has not chosen life, to do so.   It is often the case that a womb twin survivor will live out their entire lifespan without ever realising that they never chose life to the full.

There are three main reasons why a womb twin survivor may refuse life:

Ignorance: to be a womb twin survivor and remain perpetually ignorant of the fact, is to have major issues about your own existence - that somehow you don't exist, or should not exist at all. Therefore a major step towards healing is to find out if you are a womb twin survivor or not. Soon you will realise that it is your twin who is no longer in existence, not you. Then you will see clearly that you are in no way to blame for that. No longer ignorant of the reasons why you find it so hard to engage in life, your whole attitude towards being alive can change for the better.

Lack of self-awareness: Some womb twin survivors are so convinced that they are invisible or somehow "not really there" that they have no idea how they appear to others. If that is your problem, then the various forms of psycho-therapy that involve feedback on your own behaviour and the impact of your actions on other people, will be of great benefit. In the end, it's a matter of believing in your real presence in this world, and recognise that your actions have consequences on the world and the people in it. When you allow yourself to engage in the normal give and take of human life, you will be more alive.

Rage: Some womb twin survivors are so filled with rage that they are not able to function in society at all. Rage turned outward to others leads inevitably to loneliness and isolation - in extreme cases to incarceration. Rage turned inwards leads to self-harm and self-hatred - in extreme cases, suicide. Rage is neither anger nor aggression - it has elements of both, of course, but above all, rage is a particular way of expressing pain. It is a natural response to being hurt.

The rage expressed by womb twin survivors is the pain of being alive, coupled with anger at God, or The Way Things Are, and sometimes anger at the lost twin for no longer being there.

Some womb twin survivors are so enraged at being here in this world, they want only to leave it and be with their twin. Yet the survival instinct is strong, so they want to die and yet they want to live.

Addictions are a way to express this conflict. An addiction is a chosen habit that will hurt you, or even kill you one day. By means of your addiction, you can risk your life and not care if you don't survive, while trying hard not to die.

The cure for rage is two-fold: forgiveness and gratitude. The desire not to live can be understood as a reasonable and rational response to the death of your twin and can be forgiven.

Gratitude comes naturally when life can be reframed as a gift and privilege, granted only to you as the sole survivor. Your twin did not have a life, and to waste it or throw it away is an act of gross ingratitude.

Choosing life

There is a useful exercise to help womb twin survivors to understand what they are doing when they don't choose life. Take two A4 pieces of paper– one for life, one for death.

Stand with one foot on each sheet.

Now put two feet on death – how does it feel with both feet in death?

"I want to be where my twin is!"

Put two feet on LIFE – how does it feel with both feet in life?

"I want to live!"

The same exercise can be done with a group, standing in a row. Use a symbol (rope, ribbon etc) to intersect life and death. One side is powerful, the other side is lifeless.

Therapists speak from experience

* *The way to eat an elephant they say, is one bite at a time. To try and unravel the real events, giving it story, gives structure to the vagueness of the imprint, so that it can be digested in bites, in this attempt to eat the biggest elephant of all elephants. Sitting in the sacred space of the womb with others, as they remember and process the repressed trauma, is indeed a necessary and privileged step towards letting it go.*

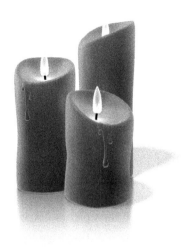

Ritual

The pre-natal memory/imprint is pre-verbal. There are many aspects of the womb twin work that cannot be achieved with words, or even conscious thought. Therefore the use of ritual is an essential element of the work. There are many kinds of ritual, and the most effective for womb twin survivors are concerned with memorial, release, re-integration and honouring.

Ritual space

A space is designated within which the ritual will be carried out. It is best if the space is private and large enough for easy movement. The size depends on the number of people involved. It can be outside or indoors. On the whole, the therapy room is not a suitable space for a ritual.

Some rituals require mood-enhancing music. Items such as cloths, stones, boxes, furniture may need to be assembled, either by the therapist or by the client. Others require access to one or more of the four elements - water, fire, air, earth.

The role of the therapist

The role of the therapist is to recommend a particular ritual where one may seem timely. If required, they may help the client in planning or carrying out the ritual. Occasionally, the therapist is asked by the client to be present when the ritual is carried out. Depending on the professional model that the therapist has adopted with this client, this may or may not be appropriate.

Three kinds of ritual

The rituals that womb twin survivors find most useful fall into three groups: expressing twin-ship, letting go and the progress of healing. The term "ritual" normally describes a prescribed series of actions, but during these rituals the womb twin survivor is allowed creative control over how things are to be done.

1. Expressing twin-ship

This kinds of ritual is centred around pairs or doubles. In drama therapy the group can re-enact the story of the Gemini twins, Castor and Pollux.

By fixing an area within the ritual space where the missing twin "resides" (e.g.. an object, empty chair etc.) the client can dialogue with the twin by entering and leaving the twin's place, or by writing a letter to the twin and then creating a reply, as it were from the twin.

The ritual space can be divided into two by means of

a long bolt of cloth, various scarves or a rope. One side can be designated the Alpha space, the other side the Beta space. The basic ritual consists of moving from one space to another.

> *To grow means to let go of the old ways and embrace the new learning. It is trust in action, stepping out of the comfort zone over and over, losing the familiar to grow, I can only grow through letting go, through losing that which was me. Life is about cycles of growth, I choose to go with the flow if life and grow with it as it teaches me.* [1]

2. Letting go

The time comes on every healing journey when it is time to let go of the past in order to move forward. The womb twin survivor can create a farewell ritual in the form of a funeral, for it's time for them to stop keeping their twin alive in their life. There have been many reports of farewell rituals - some very simple, some more complex - that have had a sudden, profound and long-lasting effect on the life of the womb twin survivor. It would seem that a ritual of letting go brings about an almost magical "cure."

As a result, some womb twin survivors are in such a hurry to get to the point of letting go, that they miss out on some of the therapeutic work that must be done first. If the ritual is carried out too soon, it will only have to be repeated later. It will not be so powerful next time.

(1) McCabe E., (2014) *Open*

Alternatively, the idea of "letting go" may feel too much like being permanently separated from the lost twin and being left absolutely alone. It may sum up images of the twin "going away" far too soon, after having "just arrived" in their awareness.

There are many womb twin survivors who find strength in their twin-ship and have no wish for a farewell ritual. This should not be taken as resistance or failure, for the likelihood is that these womb twin survivors were once half of a one-egg pair, and their needs are very different from the sole survivors of two-egg twins.

3. Reintegration

For the one-egg twins, a ritual can help to take them from feeling like "half a twin" to recognising that fact that they are, and always have been, a whole individual in their own right, even though they were parted from their other half.

The process for them is one of re-integration, and requires a ritual object made up of two very similar parts, which can be separated and brought together into a single whole.

This is an uncommon kind of object, but nevertheless, such things are often found in the home of a womb twin survivor. As the therapist, you may like to encourage your client to go home and take a good look. The chances are that they will find a suitable double object. If not they can be encouraged to look around until the right object is found.

The nature of the ritual will vary between individuals. Essentially, the object can be split to act out the initial separation when the zygote first divided, and brought together again to represent the inviolable twin bond.

The progress of healing

A healing path ritual can be created that will enable an individual - or group who meet regularly - to discover and celebrate the stage of healing they have reached.

A large ritual space is needed, with a pathway marked out. At one end is the start point - the Black Hole, which can be marked with several black cloths. At the other is the end point - usually a table, on which objects can be placed and under which inflated balloons or written messages can be hidden.

Along the path various items can be scattered, that can be chosen and used by each person as makes their healing journey, such as:

- Pink scarf for female energy, blue scarf for male energy
- Heavy stones for unforgiven hurts
- A small box for other people's pain
- Inflated balloons for messages or healing intentions
- Paper for images or messages to the lost twin

Some more ideas

Rituals can be used to make a good ending for the therapist and the client.

Other creative props include: big cuddly toys, a rolled blanket to represent the twin, teddy bears, teddy bears with a heartbeat, hot water bottle in a blanket. Young children given a teddy bear and told it is their lost twin become calmer and sleep better.

It can be helpful to hold objects that make the twin real. It is possible to obtain sets of 12-week plastic foetuses. These can be used to recreate the womb story. Russian art dolls that nest within each other can be used to represent a chimera or parasitic twin.

Different rituals are needed for two-egg vs. one-egg twins. Rituals can be carried out for each of multiples when the time is right.

A drawing or painting can be made to represent any part of the story. It can be burned as a cremation.

Use of all the elements – earth to bury; fire to burn; air to fly; water to float away or sink.

Help client to recognise that only the energy/soul of the survivor is left, not the twin's energy/soul.

Chimera – Enable the client to forgive the absorbed twin for not staying as a separate person.

Therapists speak from experience

- *The elder recommended a memorial feast. This helped the clients enormously. Just being aware of the issues of being a womb twin survivor was huge for clients. They understood the unique feelings of "something/someone missing, feeling alone and different, etc." It normalised it for the clients.*

- *Now as a writer, presenter and workshop facilitator, I ponder on ways to communicate about womb twin implications, and also inner healing methods to facilitate a process for individuals to go much deeper than most current knowledge and practice allows, to find the roots to their pain and restore order, so the fruits of their beliefs and behaviours can be altered to bring freedom and a revitalised life.*

- *It is important to really teach them to address and cope with the feelings of something missing, feeling different. Connecting with other womb twin survivors is very helpful. Having a way to acknowledge the lost twin was very helpful for clients. My experience is that most also suffer from survivors guilt and that needs to be addressed.*

- *That forgiveness is a decision you make to become free, and the feelings will develop later, is a fundamental principle of Christian Inner Healing ministries. You don't wait until you feel like forgiving. This does not excuse the one who wronged you, but separates the person from the behaviour. With parents, we can honour their position as biological parents, but not honour their behaviour when it was abusive/absent/hurtful. We can forgive and honour the twin who abandoned us.*

- *For some years now, it has become a usual thing to hold an annual baby memorial service in Christian churches or cathedrals. These services are intended for parents who have lost a baby in pregnancy or around birth, and it would not take much adapting to create a similar memorial service for womb twin survivors to remember and honour their womb twin.*

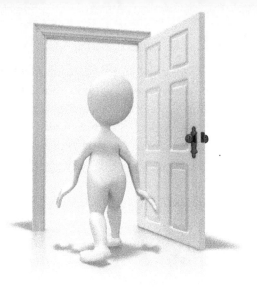

Resolution

The moment comes, when the time is right, to decide to let the healing come. But for some clients that moment of resolution is a very, very long time in coming. It seems that the womb twin survivors who try their hardest to embrace life in all its fullness, are nevertheless still frozen inside and unable to make changes. This is probably due to the effects of trauma which goes back to the time in the womb.

Trauma can be described as too much, too fast, too soon. It feels like total impotence, helplessness. You feel totally numbed; live on auto pilot; not feeling emotions any more; in shock, frozen. The traumatic reaction is to keep on going without feeling pain and employ survival mechanisms.

One of the effects of trauma from very early in life in the womb, is a compulsion to repeatedly re-create the original trauma in a variety of ways, in an attempt to master it. This effect is very similar to that of post-traumatic stress disorder that follows a trauma in adult life. Post-traumatic stress is a particular kind of stress that follows injury or severe psychological shock.

The main characteristics of post-traumatic stress disorder are sleep disturbance, vivid recall of the traumatic experience, a tendency to avoid situations that triggered the initial trauma and a withdrawal from other people and the outside world. Where the original trauma lies in the unconscious as part of the womb memory/imprint, then the symptoms of PTSD may exist without any apparent cause.

Primal integration

To counteract this, there is a process of primal integration, which is effective on trauma from birth or before. (1) Womb twin survivors can benefit from this process. It involves an exploration of the deeper levels of experience - that is, our pre-natal existence. The primitive reaction to an over-whelming experience is to freeze, fly or fight. If the trauma dates from such an early stage of development that neither flight nor fighting is an option, the only reaction left is to freeze - that is, to cease developing. In this case, the womb twin survivor remains stuck at the stage when their womb twin died, which was the original trauma.

Integrating these experiences into consciousness - i.e. acknowledging them as real memories - reduces the confusion between what was then and what is now. This is a vital part of the womb twin work, and where it is missing or incomplete, it may explain why some womb twin survivors, having done the womb twin work, still are not able to make a resolution to complete the healing journey.

Emotional freedom technique

Womb twin survivors can remain traumatised through the whole of their lives, because of the nature of the pre-natal trauma that lies in their Dream of the Womb.

Pre-natal trauma can be accessed and soothed via Emotional Freedom Technique (EFT) (1) which is very helpful to hesitant clients, who may be quite reasonably afraid of re-traumatisation through working on their pre-natal material.

Therapists speak from experience

- *I would hesitate to identify someone as a Beta or an Alpha. I don't like to use those terms. It is best to put stress on the emotions that are there in the room. Focus on feeling and helping. Too much analysis is a way not to face trauma. Rational/cognitive discussions are not sufficient to touch and heal the deep existential traumas.*

- *Having spent many years working with a progressive psychiatrist, I reached the outer limits of her practice when pre-cognitive and pre-natal issues became clear. After burning out twice at work, and a PTSD diagnosis, she referred me to a specialist in trauma.*

- *During a constellation, sometimes their reactions look like they have PTSD. They want to keep control over everything, but when their twin half "appears" their body is seen to react with heart palpitations, trembling, shortness of breath, and that gives them extra anxiety.*

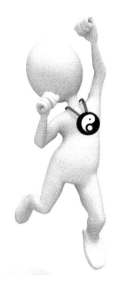

Revival

It is becoming clear, as a result of the womb twin survivors research project, that healing is possible for womb twin survivors, provided that the four main stages of the womb twin work are completed;.

Acknowledging the truth
- I am a womb twin survivor
- I have a sense of the reality of my twin's life and death

Recognising the twin bond
- I am bonded to my twin
- I want to restore that bond
- I wish to be reunited with my twin

Your self
- I am not my twin

I am a separate person with my own gifts and opportunities

Life and death

- My twin is dead and gone from this life
- I choose life for myself

How does it feel to be healed?

- A stronger sense of self
- More self control
- Greater determination to solve problems and improve personal circumstances

- Ability and courage to complain about abuse or neglect
- Preparedness to negotiate to improve relationships
- More outward focus on others, less on self
- Preparedness to help others, but now aware of the reciprocal nature of the helping relationship
- Ready to share personal story for the good of all
- Generosity of spirit but without self abnegation

The changes begin

When the work is done, changes begin:

- Difficult tasks come easier. Things are accomplished that once seemed impossible

- The client makes decisions easily, that once were overwhelmingly difficult or terrifying.

- Client feels stronger and more resilient. Workplace or playground bullying is less of a problem because the client is not prepared to act the victim any more.

- A more positive attitude towards life and being alive.

- A greater capacity for forgiveness and objectivity

- Better able to see the point of view of other people.
- Improved relationships. More open, truthful and authentic, including coming out as homosexual or bisexual.
- Able to leave therapy after making a good ending. A good ending is a good sign that the womb twin work is done. If the client simply disappears without warning or feedback, there may be more work for him or her to do at a later stage, either with you or someone else.

Finding another one

A multiple womb twin survivor (i.e. the sole survivor of triplets, quadruplets or more) may take several sessions in order to get the maximum benefit from the womb twin work.

If a client does not make a good end and keeps coming back but is not sure why exactly, then it may be time to suggest that there was more than one womb twin present.

The womb twin work is different for each womb twin, for they are all different in the way they were made and the reason why their twin died. For instance one client may have had a two-egg twin and also had a mature cystic teratoma, which was removed some years before. Another may have had an identical twin who survived almost to birth, plus a tiny foetus papyraceous, who would have been a triplet, had he or she continued to develop.

There are many hundreds of different ways in which a multiple pregnancy may be constituted. The twin bond with each womb mate needs to be explored and worked through, until the reenactment of the "Dream of the Womb" is no longer triggered by life events.

My client won't leave!

It is impossible to overestimate the strength of the twin bond among womb twin survivors, and their need to create surrogate twins in all kinds of situations.

If you have become your client's surrogate twin, he or she may love to pay handsomely for the privilege of spending an hour with you once a week, but that would not be therapy, however pleasant it might be.

Therapy would be working towards an ending, not a weekly contact to ease the loneliness of being a womb twin survivor. A client who won't leave has become dependent on you, and there are ethical considerations here: it may be great for your bank balance to make a client happy in this way, but perhaps the best therapy would be to make yourself redundant.

Therapists speak from experience

- *It is far too easy to remain stuck probing therapeutically and taking medications to manage life into a permanent grey zone.*

  - *Learning about the real power of the Spirit has provided a path of transformation where all other avenues, including endless self-help materials and training workshops, failed.*

  - *Discovery of the womb twin work connected the dots for me after many years of seeking answers through different forms of therapy. I immediately recognised its importance to my journey toward wholeness.*

Appendices

NOTE: The following pages may be copied, but for therapeuti use oly.

PROOF OF A MISSING TWIN	YES
My twin was born with me but died in the first 6 weeks of life	
My twin was born with me but was stillborn	
My twin was miscarried	
Miscarriage or suspected miscarriage but pregnancy continued	
Bleeding in the first three months	
Attempted abortion but pregnancy continued	
Mother took Clomid or other drug to stimulate ovulation	
Ultrasound evidence of a second gestational sac	
More than one embryo implanted after IVF	
Foetus papyraceous present at birth	
Additional sacs or cords found attached to placenta after delivery	
Presence of sex organs or secondary sexual characteristics of opposite sex	
Chimera (blood type or tissue)	
Dermoid cyst	
Mature cystic teratoma	
Foetus in foetu	
Split / double organs	
Additional body parts (fingers, toes etc.)	
Midline defects (spina bifida, hare lip, cleft palate, etc)	

INDICATIONS OF A MISSING TWIN	YES
Placenta unusually large	
Nodules on the placenta	
Congenital abnormality	
Left handed	
Cerebral palsy	
Mother abnormally large around the waist in the first three months	
A doctor, or nurse suspected a twin pregnancy	
A person not medically qualified suspected a twin pregnancy	
My birth was traumatic	
Breech birth	
Small for dates	
Small for dates	
There are fraternal twins among my blood relations	
There are identical twins among my blood relations	
I have always had a great interest in twins	
All my life I have had the feeling that I may have once been a twin	

Common psychological characteristics of womb twin survivors

- All my life I have felt as if something is missing
- I fear rejection
- I know I am not realising my true potential
- I feel different from other people
- I have been searching for something all my life but I don't know what it is
- Deep down, I feel alone, even when I am among friends
- I fear abandonment
- I have a problem with anger, there is too much or too little
- I always feel in some way unsatisfied, but I don't know why
- There are two very different sides to my character
- I feel restless and unsettled
- I often feel torn in two between two decisions
- I have a strong inner life, which I use as a coping mechanism
- Deep down, I feel sad all the time, even when good things are happening
- I suffer from low self-esteem

USEFUL WEB SITES

WOMB TWIN
www.wombtwin.com
High quality, well-researched information for womb twin survivors, their families and interested professionals..

WOMB TWIN SURVIVORS
www.wombtwinsurvivors.com
Althea Hayton's web site describing the womb twin survivors research project.

WREN PUBLICATIONS
www.wrenpublications.co.uk
Althea Hayton's web site with all her books about womb twin survivors. Also PDF Ebooks and Ibooks about womb twin survivors. Many of them free of charge.

VANISHING TWIN
www.vanishingtwin.com
Brent Babcock's web site with articles and details of his book, "My twin vanished, did yours?"

APPPAH
www.birthpsychology.com
Public-benefit educational and scientific organisation offering information, inspiration, and support to medical professionals, expecting parents, etc.

ISPPM
www.isppm.de
The International Society for Pre-and Perinatal Psychology and Medicine is an international, professional not-for-profit society registered in Germany

FURTHER READING

Althea Hayton, illustrated by RaRa Schlitt: *Two Little Birds*

Althea Hayton: *A Healing Path For Womb Twin Survivors*

Althea Hayton: *Womb Twin Survivors: the lost twin in the Dream of the Womb*

Althea Hayton: *A Silent Cry: Womb twin Survivors tell their Stories*

Althea Hayton: *Untwinned - perspectives on the death of a twin before birth*

Jim Cogley: *The Twinless Self (Wood You Believe 4)*

Joan Woodward: *The Lone Twin: understanding twin bereavement and loss*

Lynne Schulz: *The Survivor*

Brent Babcock: *My Twin Vanished, Did Yours?*

Elizabeth Noble: *Primal Connections*

Alfred Austermann: *The Surviving Twin Syndrome* (Original title "Das Drama im Mutterleib")

.

Lightning Source UK Ltd.
Milton Keynes UK
UKHW021543190620
365268UK00005B/840